The Latest Sirtfood Diet Beverages Cookbook

Don't miss 50 unmissable recipes to make the tastiest drinks

Anne Patel

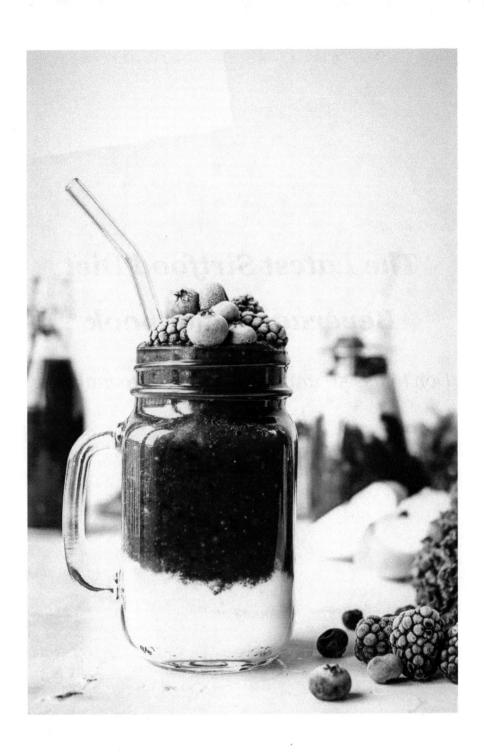

sources. Please consult a licensed professional before attempting any techniques outlined in this book.

By reading this document, the reader agrees that under no circumstances is the author responsible for any losses, direct or indirect, which are incurred as a result of the use of information contained within this document, including, but not limited to, — errors, omissions, or inaccuracies.

Table of Contents

Chapter 1: What is the Sirtfood diet

The Sirtfood Diet was created by Masters in Nutritional Medicine, Aiden Goggins and Glen Matten.

Their goal initially was to find a healthier way for people to eat, but people started losing weight quickly when they tested their program. With all the people in the world following diets hoping to lose pounds, they thought it would be selfish not to disclose their innovative health plan.

The plan they developed focuses on combining certain foods eaten in order to maximize the supply of nutrition to our body. There is an initial phase in which calories are limited to give the body a period to recover and eliminate accumulated waste. A maintenance phase follows this first phase to accustom the metabolism to the new foods you are ingesting. Throughout all stages, you will incorporate potent green juices and well-structured, well-planned meals.

The diet focuses on so-called 'sirtfoods,' plant-based foods that are known to stimulate a gene called sirtuin in the human body.

Sirtuins belong to an entire protein family, called SIRT1 to SIRT7, and each has specific health-related connections. These proteins help separate and safeguard our cells from inflammation and other damage resulting from everyday activities, helping to reduce our risk of developing major diseases, particularly those related to aging.

Studies have shown that people live longer and healthier lives when they eat diets rich in these foods that activate sirtuin, free from diabetes, heart disease, and even dementia. So this diet was designed to restore a healthy body situation, and one of the byproducts of a healthy body is also the loss of excess weight.

The diet Sirtfood is neither a miracle cure nor a week-long program designed to quickly lose weight before beach holidays. If you are only interested in losing a few pounds and then returning to your old habits, there are certainly plans and diets that are more suited to your needs.

The Sirtfood diet is a project born to help you for the rest of your life, using delicious foods, but that will also improve your health. If you switch from a standard American diet (SAD) to a sirtfood diet, you will lose all the weight your body does not need.

A healthy body does not store extra energy. It asks for what it needs and uses it effectively.

The diet isn't designed to encourage you to starve or deprive yourself. The fact is, foods that are deficient in nutrients are designer made to deprive you and, though the calories are there in plenty, your cells are still starved for the nutrition to help you thrive. The Sirtfood Diet is the opposite of deprivation and starvation. It is nourishment and balance.

Most people following the SAD may use 20 ingredients in a month, let alone enjoy the sheer volume of choice ingredients from the 120 options you will learn about here.

In recent decades, an alarming number of people have come to the conclusion that healthy food is boring, and plants or, more specifically, vegetables are terrible tasting. This is because the foods we've become dependent on – packed with sugar, salt, and unhealthy fats – have chemically altered our connection to food. Our brains are essentially lying to us, and our taste buds have been compromised.

This is one of the reasons the week-long reset is so important. After this first week, you will be able to taste food differently. The more you expose yourself to the recommended plant-based foods, the more pleasure you get out of them.

Sirtuins are critical for our health, regulating many essential biological functions, including our metabolism, which, I'm sure you know, is very closely connected to our weight. It's also a key figure in determining our body composition, such as how much muscle we build and how much fat we retain.

Sirtuin genes regulate all this and more. They're also integral in the process of aging and disease.

If we can turn these genes on, we'll be able to protect our cells and enjoy better health for longer life. Eating sirtfoods is the most effective way to accomplish this goal.

Sirtfoods are all plant-based, and they have many more benefits, in addition to being sirtuin activators.

Our bodies require energy to operate, and the majority of this fuel comes from three primary macronutrients: carbohydrates, fats, and proteins. These macros largely control our metabolic system and regulate how the calories we consume get processed by our bodies. This is why most diets focus exclusively on micronutrition and require you to calculate calories.

Our bodies need more than just energy to survive than thriving, however, which is why micronutrients are so important. They don't impact our weight as obviously as macros, but they are our health foundations.

Micronutrients, such as vitamins, minerals, fiber, antioxidants, and phytonutrients, are supposed to be consumed along with our calories. Unfortunately, in the Standard American Diet (SAD), they're in very limited supply.

When your diet is primarily made up of large quantities of red meat and processed meats, pre-packaged foods, vegetable oils, refined grains and a lot of sugar, you will have an almost total lack of micronutrition.

Plant foods offer the most micronutrients per calorie consumed. Every edible plant has a unique nutritional profile, protecting you from an innumerable variety of illnesses.

Sirtfoods, and other plant-based sources of nutrition, give your body what it needs to stay young and disease-free, and, as a bonus, this will help you remain at an ideal weight.

The original Sirtfood Diet encourages you to commit to a one week reset phase and then a 2-week maintenance phase where you rely heavily on the Sirtfood green juice for a significant dose of nutrition along with meals rich in sirtfoods. Once the phases are complete, to retain your health for the rest of your life, you will need to continue incorporating these sirtfoods into your daily meals.

The Sirtfood Diet is not a miracle cure, but if you stick to these recipes, you'll not just impress your taste buds, but you'll also enhance nearly every aspect of your health. To get safe, you don't have to count calories or starve yourself, the youthful body you've always wanted.

Sirtfood Diet Phases

Every newbie needs to understand that the sirtfood diet does not start with a single list of ingredients in your hands. Its implementation and adaptation are more than mere selective grocery shopping. Every diet can only work effectively when we allow our body to embrace the sudden shift and change in food intake. Similarly, the sirtfood diet also comes with two phases of adaptation. If a dieter successfully goes through these phases, he can continue with the sirtfood diet easily. There are mainly two phases of this diet, which are then succeeded by a third phase in which you can decide how you want to continue the diet.

Phase One

The first seven days of this diet plan are characterized as Phase One. In this phase, a dieter must focus on calorie restriction and the intake of green juices. These seven days are crucial to initiate your weight loss and usually help to lose up to seven pounds if the diet is followed properly. If you find yourself achieving this target, that means that you are on the right track.

In the first three days of the first phase, a dieter must restrict this caloric intake to 1,000 calories only. While doing so, the dieter must also have green juice throughout the day, probably three times a day. Try to drink green juice per meal. The recipes given in the book are perfect for selecting from.

Many meal options can keep your caloric intake in checks, such as buckwheat noodles, seared tofu, some shrimp stir fry, or sirtfood omelet.

Once the first three days of this diet has passed, you can increase your caloric intake to 1,500 calories per day. In these next four days, you can reduce the green juices to two times per side. And pair the juices with more Sirtuin-rich food in every meal.

Phase Two

After the first week of the sirtfood diet, then starts phase two. This phase is more about the maintenance of the diet, as the first week enables the body to embrace the change and start working according to the new diet. This phase enables the body to continue working towards the weight loss objective slowly and steadily. Therefore, the duration of this phase is almost two weeks.

So how is this phase different from phase one? In this phase, there is no restriction on the caloric intake, as long as the food is rich in sirtuins and you are taking it three times a day, it is good to go. Instead of having the green juice two or three times a day, the dieter can have juice one time a day, and that will be enough to achieve steady weight loss. You can have the juice after any meal, in the morning or in the evening.

After the Diet Phase

With the end of phase two comes the time, which is most crucial, and that is the after-diet phase. If your weight loss target has not been reached by the end of step two, then you can restart the phases all over again. Or even when you have achieved the goals but still want to lose more weight, then you can again give it a try.

Instead of following phases one and two over and over again, you can also continue having good quality sirtfood meals in this after-diet phase. Simply continue the eating practices of phase two, have a diet rich in sirtuin and do have green juices whenever possible. The diet is mainly divided into two phases: the first lasts one week, and the other lasts 14 days.

The best 20 sirt foods

All these foods include high quantities of plant compounds called polyphenols, which can be thought to modify the sirtuin enzymes, therefore, excite their super-healthy added benefits.

Top 20 sirtfoods

1. Arugula (Rocket)
2. Buckwheat
3. Capers
4. Celery
5. Chilis
6. Cocoa
7. Coffee
8. Extra Virgin Olive Oil
9. Garlic
10. Green Tea (especially Matcha)
11. Kale
12. Medjool Dates
13. Parsley
14. Red Endive
15. Red Onions
16. Red Wine
17. Soy
18. Strawberries

19. Turmeric

20. Walnuts

What Is So Great About Sirtuins?

There are seven types of Sirtuins named from **SIRT1** to **SIRT7**. Although our understanding of the exact functions of all the Sirtuins is minimal, studies show that activating them can have the following benefits:

Switching on fat burning and protection from weight gain: Sirtuins do this by increasing the mitochondrion's functionality (which is involved in the production of energy) and sparking a change in your metabolism to break down more fat cells.

Improving Memory by protecting neurons from damage. Sirtuins also boost learning skills and memory through the enhancement of synaptic plasticity. Synaptic plasticity refers to synapses' capacity to weaken or strengthen with time due to decreased or increased activity. This is important because memories are represented by different interconnected networks of synapses in the brain, and synaptic plasticity is an important neurochemical foundation of memory and learning.

Slowing down the Ageing Process: Sirtuins act as cell guarding enzymes. Thus, they protect the cells and slow down their aging process.

Repairing cells: The Sirtuins repair cells damaged by re-activating cell functionality.

Protection against diabetes: this happens through prevention against insulin resistance. Sirtuins do this by controlling blood sugar levels because this diet calls for moderate consumption of carbohydrates. These foods cause increases in blood sugar levels; hence the need to release insulin, and as the blood sugar levels increase greatly, there is a need to produce more insulin. Over time, cells become resistant to insulin, hence producing more insulin and leading to insulin resistance.

Fighting Cancers: The chemicals working as sirtuin activators affect the function of sirtuin in different cells, i.e. by switching it on when in normal cells and shutting it down in cancerous cells. This encourages the death of cancerous cells.

Fighting inflammation: Sirtuins have a powerful antioxidant effect that has the power to reduce oxidative stress. This has positive effects on heart health and cardiovascular protection.

Chapter 2: How do the Sirtfood Diet Works?

The basis of the sirtuin diet can be explained in simple terms or in complex ways. However, it's important to understand how and why it works so that you can appreciate the value of what you are doing. It is important to also know why these sirtuin rich foods help to help you maintain fidelity to your diet plan. Otherwise, you may throw something in your meal with less nutrition that would defeat the purpose of planning for one rich in sirtuins. Most importantly, this is not a dietary fad, and as you will see, there is much wisdom contained in how humans have used natural foods, even for medicinal purposes, over thousands of years.

To understand how the Sirtfood diet works and why these particular foods are necessary, we're going to look at their role in the human body.

Sirtuin activity was first researched in yeast, where a mutation caused an extension in the yeast's lifespan. Sirtuins were also shown to slow aging in laboratory mice, fruit flies, and nematodes. As research on Sirtuins proved to transfer to mammals, they were examined for their use in diet and slowing the aging process. The sirtuins in humans are different in typing, but they essentially work in the same ways and reasons.

The Sirtuin family is made up of seven "members." It is believed that sirtuins play a big role in regulating certain functions of cells, including proliferation, reproduction and growth of cells), apoptosis death of cells). They promote survival and resist stress to increase longevity.

They are also seen to block neurodegeneration loss or function of the nerve cells in the brain). They conduct their housekeeping functions by cleaning out toxic proteins and supporting the brain's ability to change and adapt to different conditions or to recuperate i.e., brain plasticity). They also help minimize chronic inflammation as part of this and decrease anything called oxidative stress. Oxidative stress is when there are so many free radicals present in the body that are cell-damaging, and by fighting them with antioxidants, the body can not keep up. These factors are related to age-related illness and weight as well, which again brings us back to a discussion of how they actually work.

You will see labels in Sirtuins that start with "SIR," which represents "Silence Information Regulator" genes. They do exactly that, silence or regulate, as part of their functions. Humans work with the seven sirtuins: SIRT1, SIRT2, SIRT3,

SIRT4, SIRT 5, SIRT6 and SIRT7. Each of these types is responsible for different areas of protecting cells. They work by either stimulating or turning on certain gene expressions or by reducing and turning off other gene expressions. This essentially means that they can influence genes to do more or less of something, most of which they are already programmed to do.

Through enzyme reactions, each of the SIRT types affects different areas of cells responsible for the metabolic processes that help maintain life. This is also related to what organs and functions they will affect.

For example, the SIRT6 causes and expression of genes in humans that affect skeletal muscle, fat tissue, brain, and heart. SIRT 3 would cause an expression of genes that affect the kidneys, liver, brain and heart.

If we tie these concepts together, you can see that the Sirtuin proteins can change the expression of genes, and in the case of the Sirtfood diet, we care about how sirtuins can turn off those genes that are responsible for speeding up aging and for weight management.

The other aspect to this conversation of sirtuins is the function and the power of calorie restriction on the human body. Calorie restriction is simply eating fewer calories. This, coupled with exercise and reducing stress, is usually a combination for weight loss. Calorie restriction has also proven across much research in animals and humans to increase one's lifespan.

We can look further at the role of sirtuins with calorie restriction and using the SIRT3 protein, which has a role in metabolism and aging. Amongst all of the effects of the protein on gene expression, such as preventing cells from dying, reducing tumors from growing, etc.), we want to understand the effects of SIRT3 on weight for this book's purpose.

As we stated earlier, the SIRT3 has high expression in those metabolically active tissues, and its ability to express itself increases with caloric restriction, fasting, and exercise. On the contrary, it will express itself less when the body has high fat, high calorie-riddled diet.

The last few highlights of sirtuins are their role in regulating telomeres and reducing inflammation, which also helps with staving off disease and aging.
Telomeres are sequences of proteins at the ends of chromosomes. When cells divide, these get shorter. As we age, they get shorter, and other stressors to the body also will contribute to this. Maintaining these longer telomeres is the key to slower aging. In addition, proper diet, along with exercise and other variables, can lengthen telomeres. SIRT6 is one of the

sirtuins that, if activated, can help with DNA damage, inflammation and oxidative stress. SIRT1 also helps with inflammatory response cycles that are related to many age-related diseases.

Calories restriction can extend life to some degree. Since this and fasting are a stressor, these factors will stimulate the SIRT3 proteins to kick in and protect the body from the stressors and excess free radicals. Again, the telomere length is affected as well.

Having laid this all out before you, you should appreciate how and why these miraculous compounds work in your favor, keep you youthful, healthy, and lean If they are working hard for you, don't you feel that you should do something too?

50 Essential Beverages Recipes

1. Matcha Green Juice

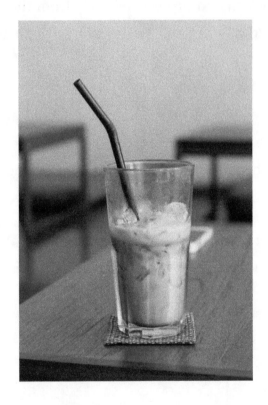

Preparation time: 10 minutes

Cooking time: 0 minutes

Total time: 10 minutes

Servings: 2

Ingredients:

5 ounces fresh kale

2 ounces fresh arugula

¼ cup fresh parsley

4 celery stalks

1 green apple, cored and chopped

1 (1-inch) piece fresh ginger, peeled

1 lemon, peeled

½ teaspoon matcha green tea

Directions:

1. Add all ingredients into a juicer and extract the juice according to the manufacturer's method.

2. Pour into 2 glasses and serve immediately.

Nutrition:

Calories: 113

Sodium: 22 mg

Dietary Fiber: 1.2 g

Total Fat: 2.1 g

Total Carbs: 12.3 g

Protein: 1.3 g

2. Celery Juice

Preparation time: 10 minutes
Cooking time: 0 minutes
Servings: 2

Ingredients:
8 celery stalks with leaves
2 tablespoons fresh ginger, peeled
1 lemon, peeled
½ cup filtered water
Pinch of salt

Instructions:
1. In a mixer, put all the ingredients and pulse until well mixed.

2. Strain the juice and pass it into 2 glasses via a fine mesh strainer.

3. Serve immediately.

Nutrition:
Calories: 32
Sodium: 21 mg
Dietary Fiber: 1.4 g

Total Fat: 1.1 g

Total Carbs: 1.3 g

Protein: 1.2 g

3. Kale & Orange Juice

Preparation time: 10 minutes
Cooking time: 0 minutes
Servings: 2

Ingredients:
5 large oranges, peeled
2 bunches fresh kale

Directions:
1. Add all ingredients into a juicer and extract the juice according to the manufacturer's method.

2. Pour into 2 glasses and serve immediately.

Nutrition:
Calories: 315
Sodium: 34 mg
Dietary Fiber: 1.3 g
Total Fat: 4.1 g
Total Carbs: 14.3 g
Protein: 1.2 g

4. Apple & Cucumber Juice

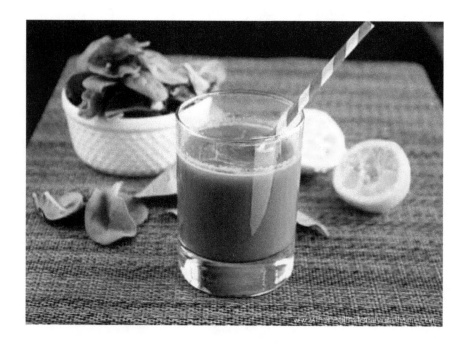

Preparation time: 10 minutes

Cooking time: 0 minutes

Servings: 2

Ingredients:

3 large apples, cored and sliced

2 large cucumbers, sliced

4 celery stalks

1 (1-inch) piece fresh ginger, peeled

1 lemon, peeled

Directions:

1. Add all ingredients into a juicer and extract the juice according to the manufacturer's method.

2. Pour into 2 glasses and serve immediately.

Nutrition:

Calories: 230

Sodium: 31 mg

Dietary Fiber: 1.3 g

Total Fat: 2.1 g

Total Carbs: 1.3 g

Protein: 1.2 g

5. Lemony Green Juice

Preparation time: 10 minutes
Cooking time: 0 minutes
Servings: 2

Ingredients:

2 large green apples, cored and sliced

4 cups fresh kale leaves

4 tablespoons fresh parsley leaves

1 tablespoon fresh ginger, peeled

1 lemon, peeled

½ cup filtered water

Pinch of salt

Directions:

1. In a mixer, put all the ingredients and pulse until well mixed.

2. Via a fine mesh strainer, drain the juice and transfer it into 2 jars.

3. Serve immediately.

Nutrition:

Calories: 196

Sodium: 21 mg

Dietary Fiber: 1.4 g

Total Fat: 1.1 g

Total Carbs: 1.6 g

Protein: 1.5 g

6. Creamy Strawberry & Cherry Smoothie

Preparation Time: 10 minutes

Cooking Time: 15 minutes

Servings: 1

Ingredients:

3½ ounces of strawberries

3.5 ounces of frozen pitted cherries

1 tablespoon plain full-fat yogurt

6.5 ounces of unsweetened soya milk

Directions:

1. Place the ingredients into a blender, then process until smooth.

2. Serve and enjoy.

Nutrition:

Calories: 203

Sodium: 23 mg

Dietary Fiber: 1.4 g

Total Fat: 3.1 g

Total Carbs: 12.3 g

Protein: 1.7 g

7. Matcha Green Tea Smoothie

Preparation Time: 3 minutes

Cooking time: 0 minute

Serves: 2

Ingredients:

2 ripe bananas 2

2 teaspoons matcha green tea powder

2 teaspoons honey

1/2 teaspoon vanilla bean paste (not extract) or a small scrape of the seeds from a vanilla pod

250 ml of milk

Six ice cubes

Directions:

1. Blend all the ingredients in a mixer and serve in two glasses.

Nutrition:

Calories: 183

Sodium: 26 mg

Dietary Fiber: 1.4 g

Total Fat: 2.1 g

Total Carbs: 12.1 g

Protein: 1.2 g

8. Green Tea Smoothie

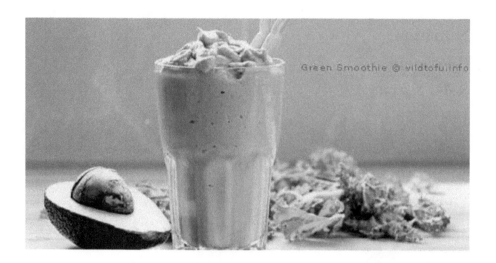

Green Smoothie @ wildtofu.info

Preparation time: 10 minutes

Cooking time: 0 minutes

Servings: 1

Ingredients:

1 ripe large banana

Milk

¼ teaspoon vanilla bean paste

3 ice cubes

1 teaspoon honey

Direction

1. In a mixer, blend all the ingredients together and serve in a glass.

Nutrition:

Calories: 185

Sodium: 21 mg

Dietary Fiber: 1.3 g

Total Fat: 2.1 g

Total Carbs: 10.3 g

Protein: 1.2 g

9. Chocolate Balls

Preparation Time: 10 minutes

Cooking Time: 15 minutes

Servings: 1

Ingredients:

2 ounces of peanut butter or almond butter

1 ounce of cocoa powder

1 ounce of desiccated shredded coconut

1 tablespoon honey

1 tablespoon cocoa powder for coating

Directions:

1. Mix all ingredients into a bowl. Scoop out a little of the mixture and shape it into a ball.

2. Roll the ball in a little cocoa powder and set aside.

3. Repeat for the remaining mixture. It can be consumed immediately or kept in the fridge.

Nutrition:

Calories: 295

Sodium: 24 mg
Dietary Fiber: 1.4 g
Total Fat: 4.1 g
Total Carbs: 16.3 g
Protein: 1.3 g

10. Strawberry & Citrus Blend

Preparation Time: 10 minutes
Cooking Time: 15 minutes
Servings: 1

Ingredients:

3 ounces of strawberries

1 apple, cored

1 orange, peeled

½ avocado, peeled and de-stoned

½ teaspoon matcha powder

Juice of 1 lime

Directions:

1. Place ingredients into a blender with enough water to cover them and process until smooth.

Nutrition:

Calories: 124

Sodium: 31 mg

Dietary Fiber: 1.4 g

Total Fat: 2.1 g

Total Carbs: 12.2 g

Protein: 1.2 g

11. Turmeric Tea

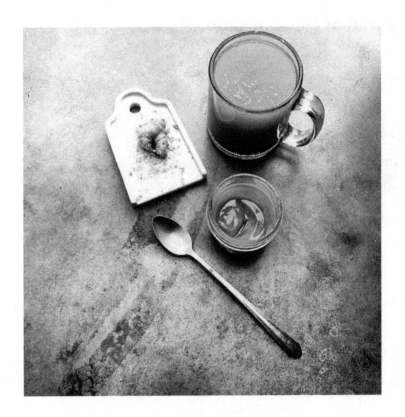

Preparation time: 10 minutes

Servings: 1

Ingredients:

1 ½ heaped teaspoon turmeric powder

½ tablespoon fresh ginger, grated

1 small lemon

Orange zest

1 teaspoon honey.

Directions

1. Boil 200ml of water in the kettle

2. In a teapot or jug, place the turmeric, ginger, and orange zest. Pour the boiling water over and quit to stand for 5 minutes.

3. Strain into a cup through a sieve or tea strainer, add lemon juice or a lemon slice and sweeten with honey.

Nutrition:

Calories: 83

Sodium: 21 mg

Dietary Fiber: 1.4 g

Total Fat: 1.1 g

Total Carbs: 1.3 g

Protein: 1.2 g

12. Strawberry and Blackcurrant Jelly

Preparation time: 10 minutes
Cooking time: 0 minute
Servings: 2

Ingredients:
Strawberries, hulled and chopped Blackcurrants washed and stalks removed
Water
3 tablespoons granulated sugar.
4 gelatin leaves

Directions:
1. Arrange the strawberries in 4 serving dishes.

2. To soften the gelatin leaves, place them in a bowl of cold water.

3. In a small pan with sugar and 200ml of water, put the blackcurrants and simmer. For 5 minutes, boil vigorously and then remove from the flame. Leave for 2 minutes to stand

4. Squeeze out the gelatin leaves with extra water and apply them to the blackcurrant mixture. Stir until it is fully dissolved, then stir in the remaining water.

5. Pour the liquid into the dishes that are prepared and refrigerate until set.The jelly should be ready in about 3 to 4 hours or you can leave it overnight.

Nutrition:

Calories: 232

Sodium: 24 mg

Dietary Fiber: 1.4 g

Total Fat: 2.1 g

Total Carbs: 10.3 g

Protein: 1.2 g

13. Green Juice Salad

Preparation time: 10 minutes

Cooking time: 0 minute

Servings: 1

Ingredients:

2 handfuls of chopped kale

1 handful of chopped arugulas

1 tablespoon chopped parsley

2 stalks of celery, sliced into bite-sized pieces ½ green apple, chopped into bite-sized pieces 6 walnuts, crushed

1 tablespoon olive oil

½ lemon, juiced

1 teaspoon grated ginger

A pinch of salt and pepper

Directions:

1. To complete this recipe, you will need to do the following:

2. Mix the juice of the lemon, ginger, seasonings, and olive oil into a small jar or small Tupperware container. Put it aside until it's ready to feed.

3. Add your kale, arugula, parsley, celery, apple, and walnut to a big bowl or large Tupperware jar. When you are ready to eat, mix it up until well mixed and set aside.

4. Shake up the dressing until you are ready to eat it, then apply it to the bowl and mix it thoroughly.

Nutrition:
Calories: 385
Sodium: 32 mg
Dietary Fiber: 1.2 g
Total Fat: 4.1 g
Total Carbs: 12.3 g
Protein: 1.3 g

14. Sirtfood Smoothie

Preparation time: 10 minutes

Cooking time: 0 minutes

Servings: 2

Ingredients:

3 ounces of plain Greek yogurt (or vegan alternative, such as soy or coconut yogurt)

6 walnut halves

10 medium strawberries, hulled

A handful of kale stalks removed

1 ounce of dark chocolate (85 percent cocoa solids)

1 Medjool date, pitted

1/2 teaspoon ground turmeric

1 small size chili

7/8 cup (200ml) unsweetened almond milk.

1 teaspoon honey

Directions:

1. Blend all the ingredients in a blender until smooth and serve in a glass.

Nutrition:

Calories: 162,

Sodium: 28 mg,

Dietary Fiber: 1.4 g,

Total Fat: 3.1 g,

Total Carbs: 11.3 g,

Protein: 1.2 g.

15. Centrifuged Green Juice

Preparation time: 10 minutes
Cooking time: 0 minutes
Servings: 2

Ingredients:

1.3 ounce of kale

1.5 ounce of rocket salad

0.7 ounce of parsley

5 ounces of green celery with the leaves

1/2 green apple

1/2 lemon juice

1/2 teaspoon of matcha tea

Directions:

1. Centrifuge the kale, rocket salad and parsley; add grated celery and apple; enrich with half a squeezed lemon and half a teaspoon of matcha tea.

2. Drink immediately so as not to lose the beneficial effects of vegetables and not keep it in the fridge. It should always be prepared when consuming it.

Nutrition:

Calories: 150

Sodium: 32 mg

Dietary Fiber: 1.4 g

Total Fat: 2.1 g

Total Carbs: 7.3 g

Protein: 1.2 g

16. Iced Cranberry Green Juice

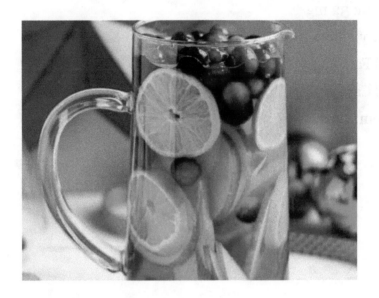

Preparation time: 10 minutes

Cooking time: 30 minutes

Servings: 1

Ingredients:

5fl Oz light cranberry juice

3½fl Oz green tea, cooled

Squeeze of lemon juice

A handful of crushed ice (optional)

Sprig of mint

Directions:

1. Pour the green tea and cranberry into a glass and add a squeeze of lemon juice.

2. Top it off with some ice and garnish with a mint leaf.

Nutrition:

Calories: 14

Sodium: 23 mg

Dietary Fiber: 1.4 g

Total Fat: 2.1 g

Total Carbs: 1.3 g

Protein: 1.2 g

17. Ginger & Turmeric Juice

Preparation time: 10 minutes
Cooking time: 7 minutes
Servings: 1

Ingredients:

1-inch chunk fresh ginger root, peeled

¼ teaspoon turmeric

1 teaspoon of honey (optional)

Ice

Directions

1. Make incisions in the piece of root ginger, without cutting all the way through.

2. Place the ginger and turmeric in a cup and pour in boiling water. Allow it to steep for 7 minutes.

3. Apply a teaspoon of honey if you wish. Let it cook and then add ice and enjoy it.

Nutrition:

Calories: 33

Sodium: 22 mg

Dietary Fiber: 1.6 g

Total Fat: 1.1g

Total Carbs: 1.3 g

Protein: 1.2 g

18. Orange & Kale Juice

Preparation Time: 10 minutes
Servings: 2

Ingredients:
5 oranges, peeled 2 cups fresh kale

Directions:
Add all ingredients into a juicer and extract the juice according to the manufacturer's method.

In case you don't have one, add all the ingredients in a blender and pulse until well combined.

Filter the juice and pass it into two glasses via a fine mesh strainer.

Serve immediately.

Nutrition Facts:
Calories 52 kcal, Fat 0.7 g, Carbohydrate 8.5 g, Protein 1.5 g

19. Spinach Smoothie

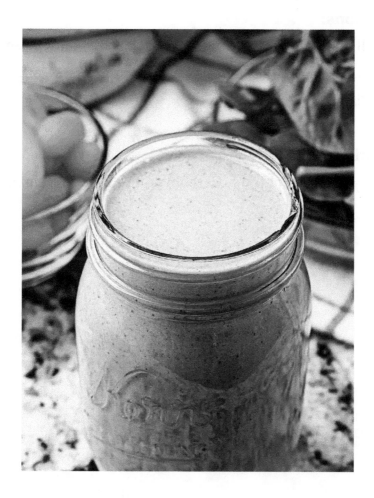

Preparation Time: 5 minutes

Servings: 1

Ingredients:

1 cup spinach

1 pear

½ bananas ¼ zucchini

½ cup almond milk, unsweetened

Directions:

Add all ingredients in a high-power blender and pulse until smooth. Pour the smoothie into two glasses and serve immediately.

Nutrition Facts:

Calories 123kcal, Fat 0.9 g, Carbohydrate 18.5 g, Protein 2.4 g

20. Lemony Apple & Kale Juice

Preparation Time: 10 minutes
Servings: 2

Ingredients:

2 green apples, cored and sliced 4 cups fresh kale leaves

4 tbsp. fresh parsley leaves 1 tbsp. fresh ginger, peeled 1 lemon, peeled

½ cup filtered water Pinch of salt

Directions:

Add all ingredients into a juicer and extract the juice according to the manufacturer's method.

In case you don't have one, add all the ingredients in a blender and pulse until well combined.

Filter the juice and pass it into two glasses via a fine mesh strainer. Serve immediately.

Nutrition Facts:

Calories 55kcal, Fat 0.3 g, Carbohydrate 6.9 g, Protein 1.2 g

21. Apple & Celery Juice

Preparation Time: 10 minutes

Servings: 2

Ingredients:

4 large green apples, cored and sliced 4 large celery stalks

1 lemon, peeled

Directions:

Add all ingredients into a juicer and extract the juice according to the manufacturer's method.

In case you don't have one, add all the ingredients in a blender and pulse until well combined. Filter the juice and pass it into two glasses via a fine mesh strainer.. Serve immediately.

Nutrition Facts:

Calories 62kcal, Fat 0.6 g, Carbohydrate 6.7 g, Protein 1.8 g

22. Apple, Orange & Broccoli Juice

Preparation Time: 10 minutes

Servings: 2

Ingredients:

2 broccoli stalks, chopped

2 large green apples, cored and sliced 3 oranges, peeled - 4 tbsp. fresh parsley

Directions:

Add all ingredients into a juicer and extract the juice according to the manufacturer's method.

In case you don't have one, add all the ingredients in a blender and pulse until well combined.

Filter the juice and pass it into two glasses via a fine mesh strainer.

Serve immediately.

Nutrition Facts:

Calories 82kcal, Fat 0.3 g, Carbohydrate 8.5 g, Protein 2 g

23. Apple, Grapefruit & Carrot Juice

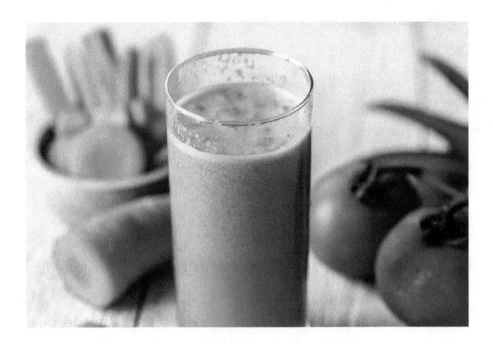

Preparation Time: 10 minutes

Servings: 2

Ingredients:

3 cups fresh kale

2 large apples, cored and sliced

2 medium carrots, peeled and chopped

2 medium grapefruit, peeled and sectioned 1 tsp fresh lemon juice

½ cup filtered water

Directions:

Add all ingredients into a juicer and extract the juice according to the manufacturer's method. In case you don't have one, add all the ingredients in a blender and pulse until well combined. Filter the juice and pass it into two glasses via a fine mesh strainer. Serve immediately.

Nutrition Facts:

Calories 67kcal, Fat 0.2 g, Carbohydrate 8 g, Protein 0.8 g

24. Fruity Kale Juice

Preparation Time: 10 minutes

Servings: 2

Ingredients:

2 large green apples, cored and sliced 2 large pears, cored and sliced

3 cups fresh kale leaves 3 celery stalks

1 lemon, peeled

½ cup filtered water

Directions:

Add all ingredients into a juicer and extract the juice according to the manufacturer's method.

In case you don't have one, add all the ingredients in a blender and pulse until well combined.

Filter the juice and pass it into two glasses via a fine mesh strainer.

Serve immediately.

Nutrition Facts:

Calories 65kcal, Fat 0.3 g, Carbohydrate 5.9 g, Protein 2.5 g

25. Green Fruit Juice

Preparation Time: 10 minutes

Servings: 2

Ingredients:

3 large kiwis, peeled and chopped

3 large green apples, cored and sliced 2 cups seedless green grapes

2 tsp fresh lime juice

½ cup filtered water

Directions:

Add all ingredients into a juicer and extract the juice according to the manufacturer's method.

In case you don't have one, add all the ingredients in a blender and pulse until well combined.

Filter the juice and pass it into two glasses via a fine mesh strainer. Serve immediately.

Nutrition Facts:

Calories 105kcal, Fat 0.5 g, Carbohydrate 12.5 g, Protein 1 g

26. Apple & Carrot Juice

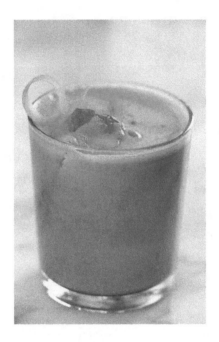

Preparation Time: 10 minutes

Servings: 2

Ingredients:

5 carrots, peeled and chopped

1 large apple, cored and chopped

1 ½-inch piece fresh ginger, peeled and chopped

½ of lemon

½ cup filtered water

Directions:

Add all ingredients into a juicer and extract the juice according to the manufacturer's method.

In case you don't have one, add all the ingredients in a blender and pulse until well combined.

Filter the juice and pass it into two glasses via a fine mesh strainer.

Serve immediately.

Nutrition Facts:

Calories 125kcal, Fat 0.3 g, Carbohydrate 21.4 g Protein 1.7 g

27. Strawberry Juice

Preparation Time: 10 minutes

Servings: 2

Ingredients:

2½ cups fresh ripe strawberries, hulled 1 apple, cored and chopped 1 lime, peeled

Directions:

Add all ingredients into a juicer and extract the juice according to the manufacturer's method.

In case you don't have one, add all the ingredients in a blender and pulse until well combined.

Filter the juice and pass it into two glasses via a fine mesh strainer. Serve immediately. It can be stored in an acceptable container for up to 3 days in the refrigerator.

Nutrition Facts:

Calories 108kcal, Fat 0.8 g, Carbohydrate 18.5 g, Protein 1.6 g

28. Chocolate and Date Smoothie

Preparation Time: 10 minutes

Servings: 2

Ingredients:

4 Medjool dates, pitted 2 tbsp. cacao powder

2 tbsp. flaxseed

1 tbsp. almond butter 1 tsp vanilla extract ¼ tsp ground cinnamon

1½ cups almond milk, unsweetened 4 ice cubes

Directions:

Add all ingredients in a high-power blender and pulse until smooth. Pour into two glasses and serve immediately.

It can be stored in an acceptable container for up to 3 days in the refrigerator.

Nutrition Facts:

Calories 234kcal, Fat 5 g, Carbohydrate 25.5 g, Protein 6 g

29. Blueberry & Kale Smoothie

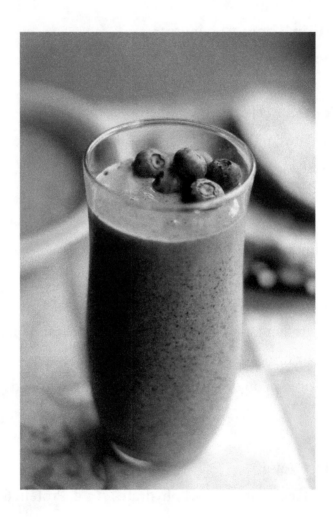

Preparation Time: 10 minutes

Servings: 2

Ingredients:

2 cups frozen blueberries 2 cups fresh kale leaves 2 Medjool dates, pitted

1 tbsp. chia seeds

1 ½-inch piece fresh ginger, peeled and chopped 1½ cups almond milk, unsweetened

Directions:

In a high-power blender, add all the ingredients and pulse until smooth. In two glasses, pour the smoothie and serve immediately.

It can be stored in an acceptable container for up to 3 days in the refrigerator.

Nutrition Facts:

Calories 230kcal, Fat 4.5 g, Carbohydrate 28.8 g, Protein 5.6 g

30. Strawberry & Beet Smoothie

Preparation Time: 10 minutes

Servings: 2

Ingredients:

2 cups frozen strawberries, pitted and chopped 2/3 cup frozen beets, chopped

1 ½-inch piece ginger, chopped

1 ½-inch piece fresh turmeric, chopped (or 1 tsp turmeric powder) ½ cup fresh orange juice

1 cup almond milk, unsweetened

Directions:

Add all ingredients in a high-power blender and pulse until smooth. Pour the smoothie into two glasses and serve immediately.

It can be stored in an acceptable container for up to 3 days in the refrigerator.

Nutrition Facts:

Calories 130kcal, Fat 0.2g, Carbohydrate 22.5 g, Protein 2 g

31. Green Pineapple Smoothie

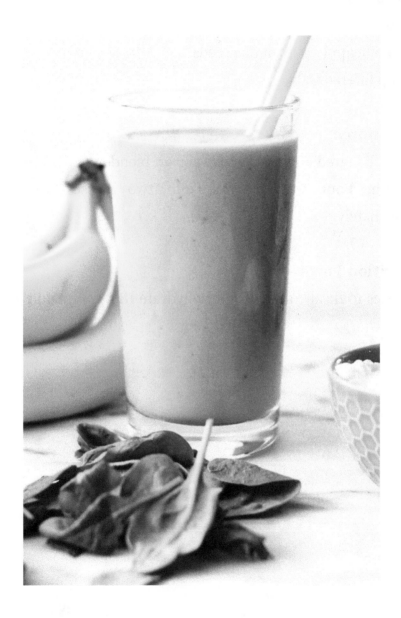

Preparation Time: 5 minutes
Servings: 1

Ingredients:

1 cup spinach

1 apple

1 cup pineapple 1tsp. of flax seeds

½ cup filtered water

Directions:

Add all ingredients in a high-power blender and pulse until smooth. Pour the smoothie into two glasses and serve immediately.

Nutrition Facts:

Calories 102kcal, Fat 0.3 g, Carbohydrate 18.5 g, Protein 1 g

32. Kale Smoothie

Preparation Time: 5 minutes

Servings: 1

Ingredients:

1 cup kale

½ mango

½ banana

1 tbsp. chia seeds

¼ cup coconut milk, unsweetened ½ cup filtered water

Directions:

Add all ingredients in a high-power blender and pulse until smooth. Pour the smoothie into two glasses and serve immediately

Nutrition Facts:

Calories 156kcal, Fat 4.5 g, Carbohydrate 20.5 g, Protein 3.2 g

33. Lettuce Smoothie

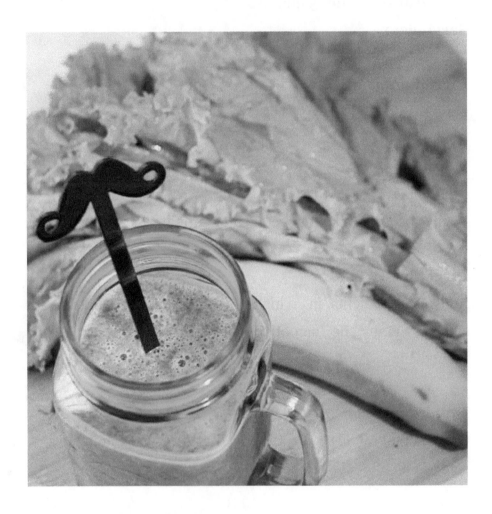

Preparation Time: 5 minutes

Servings: 1

Ingredients:

½ small head of lettuce 3 fresh plums, seeded

½ banana

1 tbsp. linseed ½ cucumber

½ cup almond milk, unsweetened

Directions:

Add all ingredients in a high-power blender and pulse until smooth. Pour the smoothie into two glasses and serve immediately.

Nutrition Facts: Calories 138kcal, Fat 2.5 g, Carbohydrate 19.8 g, Protein 3g

34. Chocolate strawberry milk

Preparation time: 5 minutes

Cooking time: 0 minutes

Serving: 1

Ingredients:

150 g strawberries, peeled and halved

1 tbsp cocoa powder (100 percent cocoa)

10 g pitted Medjool dates

10 g walnuts

200 ml milk or dairy-free alternative

Directions:

Put all ingredients in a powerful mixer and stir until smooth.

Once the matcha has dissolved, add the rest of the juice.

Nutrition:

Carbohydrates: 16

Fat: 6

Protein: 3

Kcal: 130

35. Pineapple Lassi

Preparation time: 5 minutes
Cooking time: 0 minutes
Serving: 1

Ingredients:

200 g pineapple, cut into pieces

150 g Greek yogurt

4–5 ice cubes

1 teaspoon ground turmeric

Directions:

Put all ingredients in a powerful mixer and stir until smooth.

Once the matcha has dissolved, add the rest of the juice. Just add some water and blend until you have the consistency you want, if the mixture is too thick.

Nutrition:

Carbohydrates: 13

Fat: 3

Protein: 2

Kcal: 90

36. Sirt shot

Preparation time: 5 minutes

Cooking time: 0 minutes

Serving: 1

Ingredients:

3–5 cm (10 g) turmeric root, peeled

4–6 cm (25 g) fresh ginger, peeled

½ medium-sized (70 g) apple, unpeeled Juice of ¼ lemon

Pinch of black pepper

Directions:

Put all ingredients in a powerful mixer and stir until smooth.

Once the matcha has dissolved, add the rest of the juice. Just add some water and blend until you have the consistency you want, if the mixture is too thick.

Nutrition:

Carbohydrates: 7

Fat: 10

Protein: 2

Kcal: 110

37. Hot chocolate eggnog

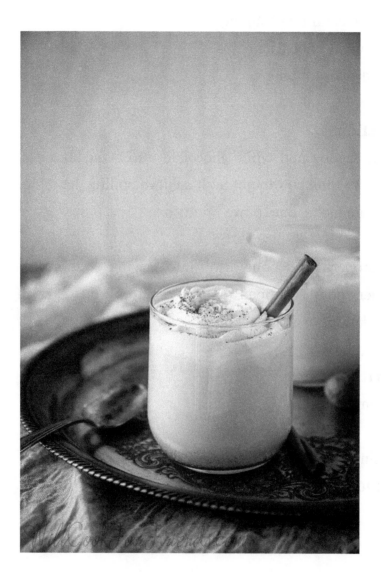

Preparation time: 5 minutes.

Cooking Time: 2 Minutes.

Servings: 4

Ingredients:
4 cups light eggnog
Whipped cream for topping
2 cups white chocolate chips
Sprinkles for topping

Directions:
Put in eggnog and white chocolate into a medium pot. Warm over low flame but do not let it achieve boiling, let it simmer till chocolate melts, one to two minutes.

Mix properly and pour drink into serving cups. In a swirling manner pour whipped cream on top and garnish using sprinkles. Have a blast!

Nutrition:
Carbohydrates: 8
Fat: 3
Protein: 1
Kcal: 100

38. Mint julep

Preparation time: 5 minutes.

Cooking Time: 15 Minutes.

Servings: 2

Ingredients:

2 tablespoon peppermint simple syrup

4 ½ cups cranberry ginger ale

4 ½ candy canes for garnish

4 ½ sprigs fresh pine for garnish

1 cup crushed ice

Directions:

Distribute peppermint syrup among the bottom of four glasses.

Put in crushed ice and pour on cranberry ginger ale. Add peppermint sprigs and candy canes in all the drinks. Have a blast.

Nutrition:

Calories: 160

Fat: 4.5g.

Carbs: 33.7g.

Protein: 1.8g.

Fiber: 0g.

39. Gingerbread latte

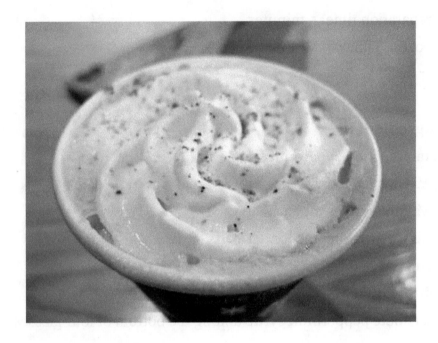

Preparation time: 10 minutes.

Cooking Time: 3 hours.

Servings: 4

Ingredients:

4 cups whole milk

3 cups brewed strong coffee

4 cinnamon sticks

1/3 cup granulated sugar

1/2 tsp ground allspice

1/4 tsp ground cloves

1 tsp nutmeg powder

Whipped cream

2 tsp ginger powder

Caramel sauce

Directions:

Mini gingerbread sweets

Put in all ingredients excluding for topping ones in a slow cooker; Mix properly.

Cover cooker: let it cook over high setting for almost three hours or over low setting for four hours.

Distribute drink among the mugs. In a swirling manner pour whipped cream on top, and then caramel sauce.

Garnish using gingerbread sweets and Have a blast!

Nutrition:

Calories: 389

Fat: 34.6g.

Carbs: 20.7g.

Protein: 4.8g.

Fiber: 0g.

40. Chili chocolate

Preparation time: 5 minutes

Cooking time: 0 minutes

Serving: 1

Ingredients:

1 chili

250 ml milk or non-dairy

Alternative 1 teaspoon cocoa powder (100 percent)

35 g dark chocolate (70 percent cocoa solids),

1 teaspoon grated date syrup

Directions:

Halve the chilies and cut into 6 or 7 pieces. Place the remaining ingredients in a small saucepan and bring to a boil over medium to high heat, stirring periodically, in order not to burn or boil the milk.

For 2-3 minutes, simmer gently, then remove from heat and leave to steep for 1 minute. Pass and serve through a fine sieve.

Nutrition:

Carbohydrates: 17

Fat: 9

Protein: 4
Kcal: 150

41. Irish coffee

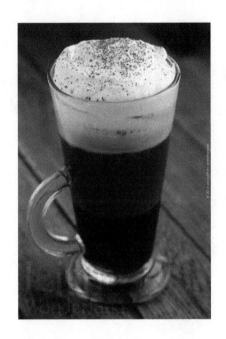

Preparation Time: 15 minutes

Cooking Time: 0 minutes

Servings: 1

Ingredients:

cl of cane sugar syrup (or 2 pieces of sugar)

2 cl of fresh cream

4 cl of coffee

3 cl of whiskey (bourbon, whiskey)

Directions:

1. Make the "Irish Coffee" recipe directly in the glass.

2. Heat the whiskey with the sugar (at low heat so as not to boil the whiskey) in a saucepan stirring. Prepare a black coffee and pour it over the hot and sweet whiskey, stir slightly. Pour everything into the formerly rinsed glass with warm water and coat the surface with lightly beaten cream, its ready! Savor without delay. To make your cream work better, place it in the freezer for 20 minutes before vigorously whipping it.

3. Despite some rumors of modern times, Irish coffee is not supposed to have the three separate floors. Other variants can be made with whipped cream instead of fresh cream, liquid cane sugar instead of powdered sugar or replace the traditional whiskey with whiskey or bourbon. Still, the original recipe is the one explained above.

4. Serve in a glass type "mug."

5. Add any grated chocolate to the cream.

Nutrition: Calories: 90 Fat: 2 g Carbohydrates: 4 g Protein: 14 g

42. Caramel coffee

Preparation Time: 15 minutes
Cooking Time: 0 minutes
Servings: 1

Ingredients:

15 cl of milk

3 cl of caramel syrup

1 dash of cinnamon syrup

1 coffee

Directions:

1. Make the recipe "Coffee Caramel."

2. Make a coffee (espresso). Heat the glass under hot water and pour the caramel syrup into the bottom of the glass. Heat the milk in another container until creamy foam and pour the warm milk gently on the syrup. Pour a few drops of cinnamon syrup and pour the coffee gently over the milk (use a spoon) until you get an extra layer...

3. Serve in a tumbler type glass.

4. Sprinkle with cinnamon powder.

Nutrition: Calories: 20 Fat: 0 g Carbohydrates: 4 g Protein: 1 g

43. Latte macchiato

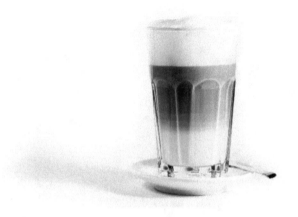

Preparation Time: 15 minutes

Cooking Time: 0 minutes

Servings: 1

Ingredients:

Coffee

20 cl of milk

Directions:

1. Make the recipe "Latte macchiato" directly in the glass.

2. Beat the milk (preferably whole) with a whisk in a saucepan over the heat to obtain foam on the surface (or using the steam nozzle of your espresso machine).

3. Pour warm milk into a heat-resistant glass (thick walls), blocking the foam with a spatula.

4. Add the milk foam on the hot milk.

5. Finally, gently pour a strong espresso (sweetened according to taste) on the frothed milk.

6. Since whole milk has a higher density than espresso, the latter will be placed above the milk.

7. Serve in a tumbler type glass.

8. To serve, you can fill the milk foam with chocolate flakes, liquid caramel, cocoa powder, cinnamon or other spices.

Nutrition: Calories: 80 Fat: 5 g Carbohydrates: 5 g Protein: 3 g

44. Latte Macchiato Caramel

Preparation Time: 15 minutes

Cooking Time: 0 minutes

Servings: 6

Ingredients:

1 l of milk

20 cl of coffee

10 cl of caramel syrup

Directions:

1. Make the recipe "Latte Macchiato Caramel" in the pan.

2. Heat the milk and prepare 20 cl of hot black coffee. Divide the milk into 4 large glasses and froth the milk with an emulsifier, electric whisk, or steam nozzle on your coffee maker until you have 2 to 3 cm of milk foam.

3. Pour about 2cl of caramel syrup into each glass and slowly pour 5cl of coffee.

4. The coffee will come just below the foam of milk, to form 3 layers: the milk at the bottom, the coffee, and the milk froth above.

5. Serve in a cup-type glass.

6. Pour a little caramel syrup over the milk foam.

Nutrition: Calories: 140 Fat: 5 g Carbohydrates: 22 g Protein: 2 g

45. Coffee Cream with Caramel Milk Foam

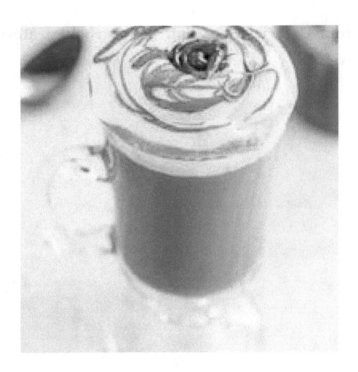

Preparation Time: 15 minutes

Cooking Time: 0 minutes

Servings: 4

Ingredients:

Grand Cru Volluto capsule (to prepare 40 ml of Espresso coffee)

100 ml of milk to prepare milk foam Teaspoon caramel syrup

25 ml / 5 teaspoons of cream (already prepared or homemade according to the method indicated below)

Ingredients for the preparation of 250 ml of homemade cream:

250 ml semi-skimmed milk

2 egg yolks

50 g of white sugar

Half vanilla pod cut lengthwise

Materials

Espresso Cup (80 Ml)

Recipe Spoon Ritual

Directions:

1. Bring the milk to a boiling point along with half a vanilla pod in a casserole dish

2. Beat the egg yolks inside a bowl with the sugar

3. Continue beating the yolks and sugar while adding the milk with the half vanilla pod

4. Then, return the mixture to the pan and allow it to thicken over low heat (do not let the mixture boil to prevent it from cutting)

5. Check the consistency of the cream with a spoon and, as soon as the cream begins to adhere to the spoon, remove the pan from the heat

6. Keep stirring the mixture to keep it soft and creamy

7. Take out the vanilla bean, scrape it with a knife to remove the seeds and put it back in the cream

8. Prepare a Volluto (25 ml) in an Espresso cup or a small Nespresso recipe glass and add 25 ml / five teaspoons of the homemade cream or ready-made cream

9. Prepare milk foam with the steam nozzle of your Nespresso machine or the Aeroccino milk frother and add the caramel syrup as soon as the foam begins to form

10. Cover the coffee cream with the caramel-flavored milk foam and serve immediately

Nutrition: Calories: 26 Fat: 1.47 g Carbohydrates: 2.91 g Protein: 0.39 g

46. Hot and Cold Vanilla Espresso with Caramel Foam and Cookies

Preparation Time: 15 minutes
Cooking Time: 15 minutes
Servings: 4

Ingredients:

For hot and cold vanilla coffee:

Two capsules of Grand Cru Volluto

A scoop of vanilla ice cream

Three tablespoons of milk foam

Two teaspoons of caramel liquid

For the cookies:

70 g softened butter

70 g of sugar

Teaspoon honey

Egg

100 g flour

A pinch of salt

50 g grated chocolate

For hazelnut caramel:

50 g whole hazelnuts

40 g of sugar

Two tablespoons of water

Directions:

1. For hot and cold vanilla coffee:

2. Prepare the milk foam, add the liquid caramel, and reserve it

3. Prepare two coffees in a large cup and pour them into a cold glass

4. Add the vanilla ice cream ball immediately and cover it with the milk foam

5. For cookies:

6. Preheat oven to 150 ° C

7. Heat sugar and water until caramelized, remove from heat and add crushed hazelnuts

8. Place the hazelnuts on a sheet of vegetable paper and roast them in the oven for 10 min, moving them occasionally

9. Put the butter, sugar, salt, honey and egg in a large bowl

10. Beat it all for a few seconds until you get a smooth mixture

11. Add caramelized hazelnuts and grated chocolate

12. Raise the oven temperature to 180 ° C

13. Put small balls of dough on the baking sheet lined with vegetable paper and bake for about 15 min

14. Let them cool on a rack

Nutrition: Calories: 190 Fat: 11 g Carbohydrates: 150 g Protein: .27 g

47. Espresso with Cottage Cheese, Lime and Brazil Nuts

Preparation Time: 5 minutes
Cooking Time: 20 minutes
Servings: 6

Ingredients:

One capsule of Grand Cru Volluto or Volluto Decaffeinato

550 g cottage cheese

100 g of sugar

The juice of a lime

Two egg whites

Three jelly sheets or a teaspoon of agar 80 g of Brazil nuts

Directions:

1. Roast the Brazil nuts in a pan and mash them finely

2. Book them

3. Dip the jelly leaves in cold water to soften them

4. Grate and squeeze the file

5. Boil 100 ml of water with sugar and lime juice for 5 minutes

6. Remove from heat and add the drained gelatin and lime zest

7. Beat the egg whites and mount them until stiff

8. Pour three-quarters of the lime syrup over the egg whites without stopping to beat and then add the cottage cheese to the mixture

9. Divide the crushed nuts into the six molds and cover them using a cottage cheese mousse

10. Pour the remaining lime syrup over and put the molds in the refrigerator for 4 hours

11. Serve it with a Grand Cru Volluto

Nutrition: Calories: 183 Fat: 5.31 g Carbohydrates: 5.5 g Protein: 27 g

48. Coffee with Malice

Preparation Time: 5 minutes
Cooking Time: 5 minutes
Servings: 4

Ingredients:
One intense espresso coffee sachet
1 splash whiskey
1 splash whole milk or cream

Directions:
1. You can use the dolce gusto machine, but if you don't have one, you can do it with a good quality soluble coffee loaded. All right; Put the coffee sachet in the coffee maker and select the amount of water to pour.

2. Activate the hot water until it stops. Have whiskey on hand.
3. Pour a little squirt of whiskey, heat a little cream or milk, and add it to coffee.

4. Ready, you can add sugar or sweetener if it's your taste. I prefer it as it is. With its bitter touch.

Nutrition: Calories: 394 Fat: 9 g Carbohydrates: 67 g Protein: 10 g

49. Viennese coffee

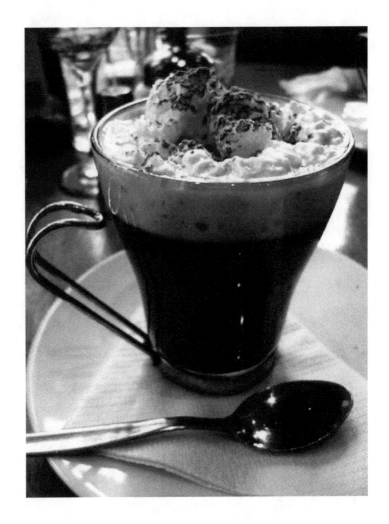

Preparation Time: 5 minutes

Cooking Time: 0 minutes

Servings: 1

Ingredients:

Espresso coffee to your liking.

Whole milk (if you are in full operation bikini... skimmed)

White sugar

Whipped cream

Shavings chocolate

Directions:

1. Take the coffee capsule. You put it in the machine and let it do its job.

2. You fill the glass of milk, add your healthy dose of sugar, and stir.

3. Decorate with a good tuft of cream and chocolate chips.

4. As you can see, very, very difficult to do. Having just spent the day.

Nutrition: Calories: 251 Fat: 27 g Carbohydrates: 0.63 g Protein: 0.62 g

50. Coffee mousse

Preparation Time: 5 minutes

Cooking Time: 0 minutes

Servings: 6

Ingredients:

4 sheets jelly

125 ml of espresso coffee

2 tablespoons. Baileys

100 gr. sugar

Two egg whites

200 ml 35% mg whipping cream

Directions:

1. We put into hydrating the gelatin.

2. We prepare a coffee.

3. We ride the egg whites with the sugar about to snow.

4. We semi-cream.

5. Melt the jello in the hot coffee and add the Baileys.

6. Add the coffee to tablespoons to the whites mounted.

7. Add the whipped cream.

8. We pour the mixture into 6 glasses that we can decorate with sprinkled cocoa powder. In my case, I prepared a coffee jelly.

9. Let cool inside the fridge for a few hours and go!

Nutrition: Calories: 2 Fat: 0.5 g Carbohydrates: 4 g Protein: 0.28 g

CPSIA information can be obtained
at www.ICGtesting.com
Printed in the USA
BVHW012329150321
602550BV00005B/616

9 781801 45686